Delicious Breakfast Chaffle Recipes

Start the Day with These Breakfast Dishes

Imogene Cook

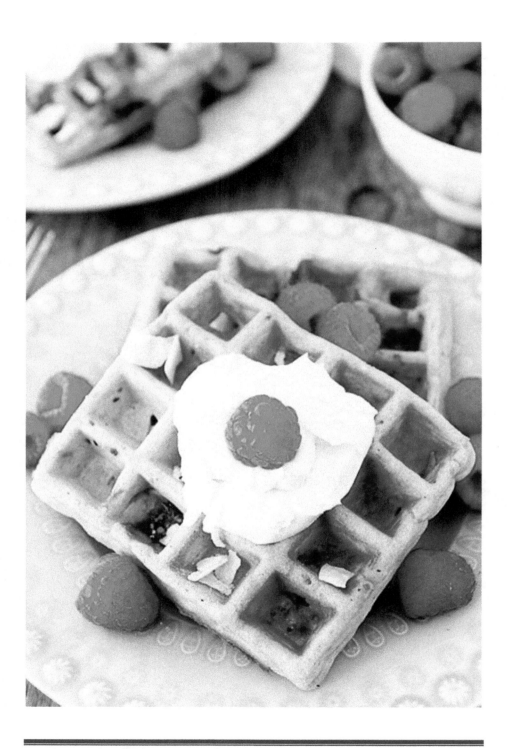

TABLE OF CONTENTS

How to Make Chaffles?

Equipment and Ingredients Discussed

Making chaffles requires five simple steps and nothing more than a waffle maker for flat chaffles and a waffle bowl maker for chaffle bowls.

To make chaffles, you will need two necessary ingredients —eggs and cheese. My preferred cheeses are cheddar cheese or mozzarella cheese. These melt quickly, making them the go-to for most recipes. Meanwhile, always ensure that your cheeses are finely grated or thinly sliced for use.

Now, to make a standard chaffle:

First, preheat your waffle maker until adequately hot.

Meanwhile, in a bowl, mix the egg with cheese on hand until well combined.

Open the iron, pour in a quarter or half of the mixture, and close.

Cook the chaffle for 5 to 7 minutes or until it is crispy.

Transfer the chaffle to a plate and allow cooling before serving.

11 Tips to Make Chaffles

My surefire ways to turn out the crispiest of chaffles:

Preheat Well: Yes! It sounds obvious to preheat the waffle iron before usage. However, preheating the iron moderately

will not get your chaffles as crispy as you will like. The best way to preheat before cooking is to ensure that the iron is very hot.

Not-So-Cheesy: Will you prefer to have your chaffles less cheesy? Then use mozzarella cheese.

Not-So Eggy: If you aren't comfortable with the smell of eggs in your chaffles, try using egg whites instead of egg yolks or whole eggs.

To Shred or to Slice: Many recipes call for shredded cheese when making chaffles, but I find sliced cheeses to offer crispier pieces. While I stick with mostly shredded cheese for convenience's sake, be at ease to use sliced cheese in the same quantity. When using sliced cheeses, arrange two to four pieces in the waffle iron, top with the beaten eggs, and some slices of the cheese. Cover and cook until crispy.

Shallower Irons: For better crisps on your chaffles, use shallower waffle irons as they cook easier and faster.

Layering: Don't fill up the waffle iron with too much batter. Work between a quarter and a half cup of total ingredients per batch for correctly done chaffles.

Patience: It is a virtue even when making chaffles. For the best results, allow the chaffles to sit in the iron for 5 to 7 minutes before serving.

No Peeking: 7 minutes isn't too much of a time to wait for the outcome of your chaffles, in my opinion.

Opening the iron and checking on the chaffle before

it is done stands you a worse chance of ruining it.

Crispy Cooling: For better crisp, I find that allowing the chaffles to cool further after they are transferred to a plate aids a lot.

Easy Cleaning: For the best cleanup, wet a paper towel and wipe the inner parts of the iron clean while still warm. Kindly note that the iron should be warm but not hot!

Brush It: Also, use a clean toothbrush to clean between the iron's teeth for a thorough cleanup. You may also use a dry, rough sponge to clean the iron while it is still warm.

Breakfast chaffle sandwich

Preparation Time: 5 minutes

Cooking Time: 15 minutes

Servings: 1

Ingredients:

- 1 egg
- 1/2 cup monterey jack cheese
- 1 tbsp almond flour
- 2 tbsp butter

Directions:

1. Preheat the waffle maker for 5 minutes until it's hot.
2. Combine monterey jack cheese, almond flour, and the egg in a bowl. Mix well.
3. Take 1/2 of the batter and pour it into the preheated waffle maker. Allow to cook for 3-4 minutes.
4. Repeat previous step for the remaining batter.
5. Melt butter on a small pan. Just like you would with French toast, add the chaffles and let each side cook for 2

minutes. To make them crispier, press down on the chaffles while they cook.

6. Remove the chaffles from the pan. Allow to cool for a few minutes. Servings.

Nutrition:

Calories: 514 Cal Total Fat: 47 g Saturated Fat: 0 g Cholesterol: 0mg Sodium: 0 mg Total Carbs: 0 g Fiber: 0 g Sugar: 0 g Protein: 21 g

Peanut butter and jelly chaffles

Preparation Time: 5 minutes

Cooking Time: 15 minutes

Servings: 1

Ingredients:

- 1 egg
- 2 slices cheese, thinly sliced
- 1 tsp natural peanut butter
- 1 tsp sugar-free raspberry
- Cooking spray

Directions:

1. Crack and whisk the egg in a small bowl or a measuring cup.
2. Lightly grease the waffle maker with Cooking spray.
3. Preheat the waffle maker.
4. Once it is heated up, place a slice of cheese on the waffle maker and wait for it to melt.
5. Once melted, pour the egg mixture onto the melted cheese.

6. Once the egg starts cooking, carefully place another slice of cheese on the waffle maker.
7. Close the lid. Cook for 3-4 minutes.
8. Take out the chaffles and place on a plate.
9. Top the chaffles with whipped cream.
10. Drizzle some natural peanut butter and raspberry on top.

Nutrition:

Calories: 337 Cal Total Fat: 27 g Saturated Fat: 0 g Cholesterol: 0mg Sodium: 0 mg Total Carbs: 3 g Fiber: 0 g Sugar: 0 g Protein: 21 g

Halloumi cheese chaffles

Preparation Time: 5 minutes

Cooking Time: 10 minutes

Servings: 1

Ingredients:

- 3 oz halloumi cheese
- 2 tbsp pasta sauce

Directions:

1. Make half-inch thick slices of halloumi cheese.
2. With the waffle maker still turned off, place the cheese slices on it.
3. Turn on the waffle maker and let the cheese cook for 3-6 minutes.
4. Remove from the waffle maker and let it cool.
5. Add low-carb pasta or marinara sauce.

Nutrition:

Calories: 333 Cal Total Fat: 26 g Saturated Fat: 0 g Cholesterol: 0mg Sodium: 0 mg Total Carbs: 2 g Fiber: 0 g Sugar: 0 g Protein: 22 g

Chaffles benedict

Preparation Time: 10 minutes

Cooking Time: 20 minutes

Servings: 4

Ingredients:

for the chaffles:

- 12 eggs
- 1 cup cheddar cheese, shredded
- 8 slices bacon

For the hollandaise sauce:

- 3 egg yolks
- 1 tbsp lemon juice
- 2 pinches kosher salt
- 1/4 tsp dijon mustard or hot sauce, optional 1/2 cup butter, salted

Directions:

1. Preheat the waffle maker.

2. Pour water in a pan and place over medium-high heat.

3. Take 4 eggs and beat them in a bowl. The remaining eggs are for poaching.

4. Once the waffle maker is heated up, sprinkle 1 tbsp of cheese and allow it to toast.

5. Take 1 1/2 tbsp of the beaten eggs and place on the toasted cheese.

6. Once the egg starts cooking, add another layer of sprinkled cheese on top.

7. Close the lid. Cook for 2-3 minutes.

8. Remove the cooked chaffle and repeat the steps until you've created 8 chaffles.

9. Fry bacon and set aside for later.

10. Poach the remaining eggs.

11. To make the sauce, combine lemon juice, salt, egg yolks, and dijon mustard or hot sauce in a bowl.

12. In a separate container, melt the butter in the microwave. Let it cool for a few minutes.

13. Pour the melted butter over the egg yolk mixture.

14. Using an immersion blender, pulse the mixture until it becomes yellow and cloudy. Continue pulsing until the consistency becomes creamy and thick.

15. To Servings, place cooked chaffles on a plate.

16. Place a slice of bacon over each chaffle.

17. Top the bacon with poached egg and drizzle with hollandaise sauce.

Nutrition:

Calories: 601 Cal Total Fat: 51 g Saturated Fat: 0 g Cholesterol: 0mg Sodium: 0 mg Total Carbs: 1 g Fiber: 0 g Sugar: 0 g Protein: 34 g

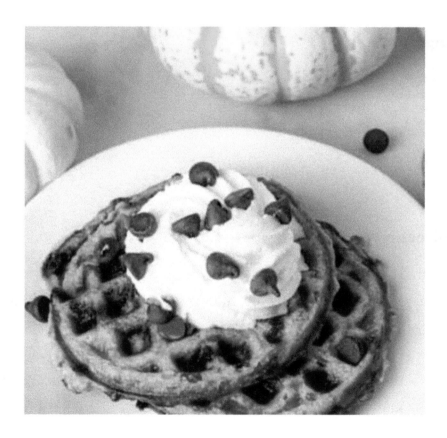

Carnivore chaffle

Preparation Time: 5 minutes

Cooking Time: 10 minutes

Servings: 1

Ingredients:

- 1 egg
- 1/3 cup mozzarella cheese
- 1/2 cup pork rinds
- Salt

Directions:

1. Preheat the waffle maker.
2. In a small mixing bowl, mix a pinch of salt with the cheese, egg, and pork rinds.
3. Pour the mixture onto the preheated waffle maker. Close the lid and wait for 3-5 minutes while it cooks. You'll know it's cooked once it already has a golden-brown color.
4. Carefully remove it from the waffle maker and Servings.

Nutrition:

Calories: 274 Cal Total Fat: 20 g Saturated Fat: 0 g Cholesterol: 0 mg Sodium: 0 mg Total Carbs: 1 g Fiber: 0 g Sugar: 0 g Protein: 23 g

Cauliflower chaffle

Preparation time: 5 minutes

Cooking time: 5 minutes

Servings: 1

Ingredients:

- 1/2 cup of rice cauliflower
- 1/4 shredded cheddar
- 1 large egg from which half of the yolk has been removed
- 1 tbsp fine almond flour
- Salt and pepper
- Sprinkle extra cheese on the bottom.

Directions:

1. spread the mix on a waffle iron and add more cheese.
2. Cook for 8 minutes.

Note: when immersed in ketchup, it tastes like a hash brown. Oh, it cuts the cheese in half

Nutrition:

Calories: 200 Cal Total Fat: 16 g Saturated Fat: 0 g Cholesterol: 0 mg Sodium: 0 mg Total Carbs: 2 g Fiber: 2 g Sugar: 0 g Protein: 11 g

Hot Dog Chaffles

Preparation Time: 15 minutes

Cooking Time: 14 minutes

Servings: 2

Ingredients:

- 1 egg, beaten
- 1 cup finely grated cheddar cheese
- 2 hot dog sausages, cooked
- Mustard dressing for topping
- 8 pickle slices

Directions:

1. Preheat the waffle iron.
2. In a medium bowl, mix the egg and cheddar cheese.
3. Open the iron and add half of the mixture. Close and cook until crispy, 7 minutes.
4. Transfer the chaffle to a plate and make a second chaffle in the same manner.

5. To serve, top each chaffle with a sausage, swirl the mustard dressing on top, and then divide the pickle slices on top.
6. Enjoy!

Nutrition:

Calories: 231 Cal Total Fat: 18.29 g Saturated Fat: 0 g

Cholesterol: 0 mg Sodium: 0 mg Total Carbs: 2.8 g Fiber: 0 g Sugar: 0 gnProtein: 13.39 g

Omelette

Preparation Time: 8 minutes

Cooking Time: 17 minutes

Servings: 2

Ingredients:

- 7 ounces of spinach (frozen)
- Half of a dozen large eggs (six)
- 2 tablespoons of milk (you should use heavy cream or almond milk)
- 2 teaspoons of oil for frying (we are going to use olive oil)
- A single tablespoon of herbs (chives or parsley is good, but you need to make sure that they are fresh)
- A quarter of a cup of grated sharp cheddar A quarter of a cup of grated parmesan cheese
- A quarter of a cup of crumbled, mild feta cheese
- A single handful of kale that is chopped (discard the stems)
- A half of a cup of ricotta cheese
- Pepper for taste

Directions:

1. Make sure that there is no liquid in your spinach. If there is, then you will need to squeeze it out. You should have a small handful left.
2. Chop the spinach finely then do the same with the kale (a food processor makes this easier and quicker).
3. Add the parmesan cheese along with cheddar, eggs, and milk and mix it well so it will combine well.
4. Mix the herbs, feta, and ricotta in a separate bowl and then season with pepper.
5. Place the bowl to the side.
6. Heat a single teaspoon of olive oil in a pan that is non-stick.
7. Pour in half of the egg mix you made.
8. On medium-high heat fry until just set.
9. Add half of the ricotta mix on top before folding the omelette over.
10. Be careful when you do this.
11. Place a lid over the pan and then cook for another minute so that your filling is warmed.
12. Repeat for the second omelette.

Nutrition:

Calories: 522 Cal Total Fat: 34.7 g Saturated Fat: 0 g Cholesterol:0 mg Sodium: 0 mg Total Carbs: 10.3 g Fiber: 2.4 g Sugar: 0 g Protein: 44 g

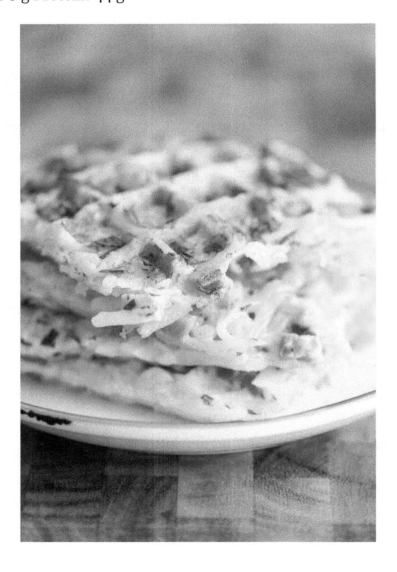

Pandan Asian Chaffles

Preparation Time: 3 minutes

Cooking Time: 8 minutes

Servings: 2

Ingredients:

- ½ cup cheddar cheese, finely shredded
- 1 egg
- 3 drops of pandan extract
- 1 tbsp almond flour
- 1/3 tsp garlic powder

Directions:

1. Warm up your mini waffle maker.
2. Mix the egg, almond flour, garlic powder with cheese in a small bowl.
3. Add pandan extract to the cheese mixture and mix well.
4. For a crispy crust, add a teaspoon of shredded cheese to the waffle maker and cook for 30 seconds.
5. Then, pour the mixture into the waffle maker and cook for 5 minutes or until crispy.

6. Repeat with remaining batter.
7. Serve with fried chicken wings with bbq sauce and enjoy!

Nutrition:

Calories: 170 Cal Total Fat: 13 g Saturated Fat: 0 g Cholesterol: 0 mg Sodium: 0 mg Total Carbs: 2 g Fiber: 0 g Sugar: 0 g Protein: 11 g

Ham and Jalapenos Chaffle

Preparation Time: 5 minutes

Cooking Time: 9 minutes

Servings: 3

Ingredients:

- 2 lbs cheddar cheese, finely grated
- 2 large eggs
- ½ jalapeno pepper, finely grated
- 2 ounces ham steak
- 1 medium scallion
- 2 tsp coconut flour

Directions:

1. Shred the cheddar cheese using a fine grater.
2. Deseed the jalapeno and grate using the same grater.
3. Finely chop the scallion and ham.
4. Pour all the ingredients in a medium bowl and mix well.
5. Spray your waffle iron with cooking spray and heat for 3 minutes.
6. Pour 1/4 of the batter mixture into the waffle iron.

7. Cook for 3 minutes, until crispy around the edges.

8. Remove the waffles from the heat and repeat until all the batter is finished.

9. Once done, allow them to cool to room temperature and enjoy.

Nutrition:

Calories: 120 Cal Total Fat: 10 g Saturated Fat: 0 g Cholesterol: 0 mg Sodium: 0 mg Total Carbs: 2 g Fiber: 0 g Sugar: 0 g Protein: 12 g

Hot Ham Chaffles

Preparation Time: 5 minutes

Cooking Time: 4 minutes

Servings: 4

Ingredients:

- ½ cup mozzarella cheese, shredded
- 1 egg
- ¼ cup ham, chopped
- ¼ tsp salt
- 2 tbsp mayonnaise
- 1 tsp Dijon mustard

Directions:

1. Preheat your waffle iron.
2. In the meantime, add the egg in a small mixing bowl and whisk.
3. Add in the ham, cheese, and salt. Mix to combine.
4. Scoop half the mixture using a spoon and pour into the hot waffle iron.

5. Close and cook for 4 minutes.
6. Remove the waffle and place on a large plate. Repeat the process with the remaining batter.
7. In a separate small bowl, add the mayo and mustard. Mix together until smooth.
8. Slice the waffles in quarters and use the mayo mixture as the dip.

Nutrition:

Calories: 110 Cal Total Fat: 12 g Saturated Fat: 0 g Cholesterol: 0 mg Sodium: 0 mg Total Carbs: 6 g Fiber: 0 g Sugar: 0 g Protein: 12 g

Bacon & Egg Chaffles

Preparation Time: 5 minutes

Cooking Time: 10 minutes

Servings: 2

Ingredients:

- 2 eggs
- 4 tsp collagen peptides, grass-fed
- 2 tbsp pork panko
- 3 slices crispy bacon

Directions:

1. Warm up your mini waffle maker.
2. Combine the eggs, pork panko, and collagen peptides. Mix well. Divide the batter in two small bowls.
3. Once done, evenly distribute ½ of the crispy chopped bacon on the waffle maker.
4. Pour one bowl of the batter over the bacon. Cook for 5 minutes and immediately repeat this step for the second chaffle.

5. Plate your cooked chaffles and sprinkle with extra Panko for an added crunch.
6. Enjoy!

Nutrition:

Calories: 266 Cal Total Fat: 17 g Saturated Fat: 0 g Cholesterol: 0 mg Sodium: 0 mg Total Carbs: 11.2 g Fiber: 0 g Sugar: 0 g Protein: 27 g

Cheese-free Breakfast Chaffle

Preparation Time: 4 minutes

Cooking Time: 12 minutes

Servings: 1

Ingredients:

- 1 egg
- ½ cup almond milk ricotta, finely shredded.
- 1 tbsp almond flour
- 2 tbsp butter

Directions:

1. Mix the egg, almond flour and ricotta in a small bowl.
2. Separate the chaffle batter into two and cook each for 4 minutes.
3. Melt the butter and pour on top of the chaffles.
4. Put them back in the pan and cook on each side for 2 minutes.
5. Remove from the pan and allow them sit for 2 minutes.
6. Enjoy while still crispy.

Nutrition:

Calories: 530 Cal Total Fat: 50 g Saturated Fat: 0 g Cholesterol: 0mg Sodium: 0 mg Total Carbs: 3 g Fiber: 0 g Sugar: 0 g Protein: 23 g

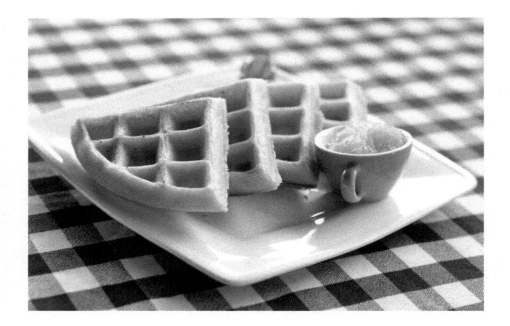

Bacon Chaffle Omelettes

Preparation Time: 5 minutes

Cooking Time: 10 minutes

Servings: 2

Ingredients:

- 2 slices bacon, raw
- 1 egg
- 1 tsp maple extract, optional
- 1 tsp all spices

Directions:

1. Put the bacon slices in a blender and turn it on.
2. Once ground up, add in the egg and all spices. Go on blending until liquefied.
3. Heat your waffle maker on the highest setting and spray with non-stick cooking spray.
4. Pour half the omelette into the waffle maker and cook for 5 minutes max.
5. Remove the crispy omelette and repeat the same steps with rest batter.

6. Enjoy warm.

Nutrition:

Calories: 59 Cal Total Fat: 4.4 g Saturated Fat: 0 g Cholesterol: 0mg Sodium: 0 mg Total Carbs: 1 g Fiber: 0 g Sugar: 0 g Protein: 5 g

Avocado Chaffle Toast

Preparation Time: 4 minutes

Cooking Time: 8 minutes

Servings: 2

Ingredients:

- ½ avocado
- 1 egg
- ½ cup cheddar cheese, finely shredded
- 1 tbsp almond flour
- 1 tsp lemon juice, fresh
- Salt, ground pepper to taste
- Parmesan cheese, finely shredded for garnishing

Directions:

1. Warm up your mini waffle maker.
2. Mix the egg, almond flour with cheese in a small bowl.
3. For a crispy crust, add a teaspoon of shredded cheese to the waffle maker and cook for 30 seconds.
4. Then, pour the mixture into the waffle maker and cook for 5 minutes or until crispy.

5. Repeat with remaining batter.

6. Mash avocado with a fork until well combined and add lemon juice, salt, pepper

7. Top each chaffle with avocado mixture. Sprinkle with parmesan and enjoy!

Nutrition:

Calories: 250 Cal Total Fat: 23 g Saturated Fat: 0 g Cholesterol: 0mg Sodium: 0 mg Total Carbs: 9 g Fiber: 0 g Sugar: 0 g Protein: 14 g

Keto Chaffle Waffle

Preparation time:

Cooking time:

Ingredients:

- 1 egg
- ½ cup of shredded mozzarella cheese
- 1 ½ table-spoon of almond flour
- Pinch of baking powder

Equipment:

- Waffle Maker
- Shredder (to shred solid mozzarella cheese)

Directions:

1. Start by turning your waffle maker on and preheating it. During the time of pre-heating, in a bowl, whisk the egg and shredded mozzarella cheese together. If you do not have shredded mozzarella cheese, you can use the shredder to shred your cheese, then add the almond

powder and baking powder to the bowl and whisk them until the mixture is consistent.

2. Then pour the mixture onto the waffle machine. Make sure you pour it to the center of the mixture will come out of the edges on closing the machine. Close the machine and let the waffles cook until golden brown. Then you can serve your tasty chaffle waffles.

Nutrition:

Serves 1 person Calories 320 Carbohydrates 2.9 g Protein 21.5 g Fat 24.3g

Keto Chaffle Topped with Salted Caramel Syrup

Preparation time: 15 mins

Cooking time: 10 mins

Ingredients:

- 1 egg
- ½ cup of mozzarella cheese
- ¼ cup of cream
- 2 tablespoon of collagen powder
- 1 ½ tablespoon of almond flour
- 1 ½ tablespoon of unsalted butter
- Pinch of salt
- ¾ tablespoon of powdered erythritol
- Pinch of baking powder

Directions:

1. Begin by preheating your waffle machine by switching it on and turning the heat to medium. Whisk together the chaffle ingredients that include the egg, mozzarella

cheese, almond flour, and baking powder. Pour the mixture on the waffle machine. Let it cook until golden brown. You can make up to two chaffles with this method.

2. To make the caramel syrup, you will need to turn on the flame under a pan to medium heat Melt the unsalted butter on the pan. Then turn the heat low and add collagen powder and erythritol to the pan and whisk them. Gradually add the cream and remove from heat. Then add the salt and continue to whisk. Pour the syrup onto the chaffle, and here you go.

Nutrition:

1 serving 605 calories 45g fat 48g protein 5.1 g of carbohydrates

Keto Chaffle Bacon Sandwich

Preparation time: 15 mins

Cooking time: 10 mins

Ingredients:

- 1 egg
- ½ cup of shredded mozzarella cheese
- 2 Tablespoon of coconut flour
- 2 strips of pork or beef bacon
- 1 slice of any type of cheese
- 2 tablespoon of coconut oil

Directions:

1. To make the chaffle, you will be following the typical recipe for making a chaffle. Start by warming your waffle machine to medium heat. In a bowl, beat 1 egg, ½ cup of mozzarella cheese, and almond flour. Pour the mixture on the waffle machine. Let it cook until it is golden brown. Then remove in a plate.
2. Warm coconut oil in a pan over medium heat. Then place the bacon strips in the pan. Cook until crispy over

medium heat. Assemble the bacon and cheese on the chaffle.

Nutrition:

Serving size 1 Calories 580 Fat 52 g Carbohydrates 3g

Crispy Zucchini Chaffle

Preparation time: 15 mins

Cooking time: 5 mins

Ingredients:

- 2 eggs
- 1 fresh zucchini
- 1 cup of shredded or grated cheddar cheese
- 2 pinch of salt
- 1 tablespoon of onion (chopped)
- 1 clove of garlic

Equipment:

- Waffle maker
- Grater to grate the cheese

Directions:

1. Start by preheating the waffle maker to medium heat. The best way to make a chaffle is to make it with layering. Start by dicing onions and mashing the garlic. Then use the grater to grate the zucchini. Then take a bowl and add 2 eggs and add the grated zucchini to the bowl.

2. 2Also, add the onions, salt, and garlic for extra flavor. You can also add other herbs to give your zaffle a crispy more flavor. Then sprinkle ½ cup of cheese on top of the waffle machine.

3. Add the mixture from the bowl to the waffle machine. Add the remaining cheese on top of the waffle machine and close the waffle machine. Make sure the waffle cooks for about 3 to 5 minutes until it turns golden brown.

4. By the layering method, you will achieve the perfect crisp. Take out your zucchini chaffles and serve them hot and fresh.

Nutrition:

Serving size 2 Calories 170 Fat 12g Carbohydrates 4g Protein 11g

Peanut Butter Chaffle

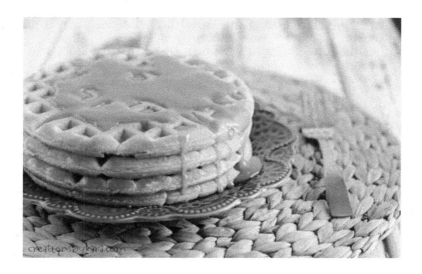

Preparation time: 15 min

Cooking time: 10 min

Ingredients:

- 1 egg
- ½ cup of cheddar cheese
- 2 tablespoon of peanut butter
- Few drops of vanilla extract

Equipment:

- Waffle maker
- Grater

Directions:

1. To make deliciously tasting peanut butter chaffles. Take a grater and grate some cheddar cheese. Add one egg, cheddar cheese, 2 tablespoon of peanut butter, and a few drops of vanilla extract. Beat these ingredients together until the batter is consistent enough.

2. Then sprinkle some shredded cheese as a base on the waffle maker. Pour the mixture on top of the waffle machine.

3. Sprinkle more cheese on top of the mixture and close the waffle machine. Ensure that the waffle is cooked thoroughly for about a few minutes until they are golden brown. Then remove it and enjoy your deliciously cooked chaffles.

Nutrition:

1 serving 363 Calories 29 g of Fat 22 g of Protein 4 g of Carbohydrates

Buffalo hummus beef chaffless

Preparation time: 15 minutes

Cooking time: 32 minutes

Servings: 4

Ingredients:

- Two eggs
- 1 cup + ¼ cup finely grated cheddar cheese, divided two chopped fresh scallions
- Salt and freshly ground black pepper to taste
- Two chicken breasts, cooked and diced ¼ cup buffalo sauce
- 3 tbsp low-carb hummus
- Two celery stalks, chopped
- ¼ cup crumbled blue cheese for topping

Directions:

1. Preheat the waffle iron.
2. In a medium bowl, mix the eggs, 1 cup of the cheddar cheese, scallions, salt, and black pepper,

3. Open the iron and add a quarter of the mixture. Close and cook until crispy, 7 minutes.

4. Transfer the chaffle to a plate and make three more chaffless in the same manner.

5. Preheat the oven to 400 f and line a baking sheet with parchment paper. Set aside.

6. Cut the chaffless into quarters and arrange on the baking sheet.

7. In a medium bowl, mix the chicken with the buffalo sauce, hummus, and celery.

8. Spoon the chicken mixture onto each quarter of chaffless and top with the remaining cheddar cheese.

9. Place the baking sheet in the oven and bake until the cheese melts, 4 minutes.

10. Remove from the oven and top with the blue

11. cheese.

12. Servings afterwards

Nutrition:

Calories: 552 Cal Total Fat: 28.37 g Saturated Fat: 0g Cholesterol: 0 mg Sodium: 0 mg Total Carbs: 6.97 g Fibre: 0 g Sugar: 0g Protein: 59.8 g

Cauliflower Turkey Chaffle

Preparation Time: 5 minutes

Cooking Time: 12 minutes

Servings: 2

Ingredients:

- One large egg (beaten)
- ½ cup cauliflower rice
- ¼ cup diced turkey
- ½ tsp coconut amino or soy sauce
- A pinch of ground black pepper
- A pinch of white pepper
- ¼ tsp curry
- ¼ tsp oregano
- 1 tbsp butter (melted)
- ¾ cup shredded mozzarella cheese
- One garlic clove (crushed)

Directions:

1. Plug the waffle maker to preheat it and spray it with a non-stick spray.
2. In a mixing bowl, combine the cauliflower rice, white pepper, black pepper, curry, and oregano.

3. In another mixing bowl, whisk together the eggs, butter, crushed garlic, and coconut amino.
4. Pour the egg mixture into the cheese mixture and mix until the ingredients are well combined.
5. Add the diced turkey and stir to combine.
6. Sprinkle 2 tbsp cheese over the waffle maker. Fill the waffle maker with an appropriate amount of the batter. Spread out the mixture to the edges to cover all the holes on the waffle maker. Sprinkle another 2 tbsp cheese over the dough.
7. Close the waffle maker and cook for about 4 minutes or according to the waffle maker's settings.
8. After the cooking cycle, use a plastic or silicone utensil to remove the chaffle from the waffle maker.
9. Repeat steps 6 to 8 until you have cooked all the batter into chaffless.
10. Serve warm and enjoy.

Nutrition:

Servings: 2 Amount per serving Calories 168 % Daily Value Total Fat 11.5g 15% Saturated Fat 6.1g 30% Cholesterol 127mg 42% Sodium 184mg 8% Total Carbohydrate 3.8g 1% Dietary Fiber 0.2g 1% Total Sugars 1.2g Protein 12.5g Vitamin D 13mcg 64% Calcium 30mg 2% Iron 2mg 13% Potassium 101mg 2%

Chaffle with Sausage Gravy

Preparation Time: 10 minutes

Cooking Time: 15 minutes

Servings: 2

Ingredients:

Sausage Gravy:

- ¼ cup cooked breakfast sausage
- 1/8 tsp onion powder
- 1/8 tsp garlic powder
- ½ tsp pepper or more to taste
- 3 tbsp chicken broth
- 2 tsp cream cheese
- 2 tbsp heavy whipping cream
- ¼ tsp oregano

Chaffle:

- 1 tbsp almond flour
- 1 tbsp finely chopped onion
- 1/8 tsp salt
- ¼ tsp baking powder
- ½ cup mozzarella cheese
- 1 egg (beaten)

Directions:

1. Plug the waffle maker to preheat it and spray it with a non-stick spray.
2. In a mixing bowl, combine the almond flour, chopped onion, mozzarella, baking powder, and salt. Add the egg and mix until the ingredients are well combined.
3. Close the waffle maker and bake for about 4 minutes or according to the waffle maker's settings.
4. After the baking cycle, remove the chaffle from the waffle maker with a silicone or plastic utensil.
5. Repeat steps 3 to 5 until you have cooked all the batter into chaffless.
6. Heat a skillet over medium to high heat. A
7. Pour in the chicken broth and add the oregano, garlic powder, onion powder, pepper, cream cheese and whipping cream.
8. Bring to a boil, reduce the heat and simmer for about 7 minutes or until the gravy sauce thickens.
9. Serve the chaffless with the gravy and enjoy it.

Nutrition:

Servings: 2 Amount per serving Calories 198 % Daily Value Total Fat 16.6g 21% Saturated Fat 7.3g 36% Cholesterol 123mg 41% Sodium 429mg 19% Total Carbohydrate 3.3g 1% Dietary Fiber 0.8g 3% Total Sugars 0.7g Protein 9.8g Vitamin D 16mcg 78% Calcium 74mg 6% Iron 1mg 6% Potassium 195mg 4%

Lobster Chaffle

Preparation Time: 5 minutes

Cooking Time: 8 minutes

Servings: 2

Ingredients:

- 1 egg (beaten)
- ½ cup shredded mozzarella cheese
- ¼ tsp garlic powder
- ¼ tsp onion powder
- 1/8 tsp Italian seasoning

Lobster Filling:

- ½ cup lobster tails (defrosted)
- 1 tbsp mayonnaise
- 1 tsp dried basil
- 1 tsp lemon juice
- 1 tbsp chopped green onion

Directions:

1. Plug the waffle maker to preheat it and spray it with a non-stick
2. cooking spray.

3. In a mixing bowl, combine the mozzarella, Italian seasoning, garlic, and onion powder. Add the egg and mix until the ingredients are well combined.
4. Pour an appropriate amount of the batter into the waffle maker and spread out the dough to cover all the holes on the waffle maker.
5. Close the waffle maker and cook for about 4 minutes or according to your waffle maker's settings.
6. After the cooking cycle, use a plastic or silicone utensil to remove and transfer the chaff to a wire rack to cool.
7. Repeat steps 3 to 5 until you have cooked all the batter into chaffless.
8. For the filling, put the lobster tail in a mixing bowl and add the mayonnaise, basil and lemon juice. Toss until the ingredients are well combined.
9. Fill the chaffless with the lobster mixture and garnish with chopped green onion.
10. Serve and enjoy.

Nutrition:

Servings: 2 Amount per serving Calories 117 % Daily Value* Total Fat 6.3g 8% Saturated Fat 1.9g 10% Cholesterol 141mg 47% Sodium 303mg 13% Total Carbohydrate 3g 1% Dietary Fiber 0.2g 1% Total Sugars 1g Protein 11.9g Vitamin D 8mcg 39% Calcium 57mg 4% Iron 1mg 3% Potassium 133mg 3%

Savory Pork Rind Chaffle

Preparation Time: 5 minutes

Cooking Time: 10 minutes

Servings: 2

Ingredients:

- ¼ tsp paprika
- ¼ tsp oregano
- ¼ tsp garlic powder
- 1/8 tsp ground black pepper or to taste
- ½ onion (finely chopped)
- ½ cup pork rind (crushed)
- ½ cup mozzarella cheese
- 1 large egg (beaten)

Directions:

1. Plug the waffle maker to preheat it and spray I with a non-stick cooking spray.
2. In a mixing bowl, combine the crushed pork rind, cheese, onion, paprika, garlic powder, and pepper. Add the egg

and mix until the ingredients are well combined.

3. Pour an appropriate amount of the batter into the waffle maker and spread out the dough to cover all the holes on the waffle maker.

4. Close the waffle maker and cook for about 5 minutes or according to your waffle maker's settings.

5. After the cooking cycle, use a plastic or silicone utensil to remove the chaffle from the waffle maker.

6. Repeat steps 3 to 5 until you have cooked all the batter into chaffless.

7. Serve and top with sour cream as desired.

Nutrition:

Servings: 2 Amount per serving Calories 392 % Daily Value*Total Fat 24g 31% Saturated Fat 9.6g 48% Cholesterol 177mg 59% Sodium 1169mg 51% Total Carbohydrate 3.6g 1% Dietary Fiber 0.8g3% Total Sugars 1.5g Protein 41.9g Vitamin D 9mcg 44% Calcium 29mg2% Iron 1mg 4%Potassium 88mg 2%

Smoked salmon

Preparation Time: 10 minutes

Cooking Time: 20 minutes

Servings: 6

Ingredients:

- 7 ounces of salmon (smoked)
- The zest from half of a lemon)
- 8 ounces of cream cheese
- 4 tablespoons of dill (fresh)
- 5 and an additional 1/3 tablespoons of mayo
- 2 ounces of lettuce

Directions:

1. Cut your salmon into small pieces.
2. Combine all of your ingredients in a bowl.
3. Let it sit for 15 minutes.
4. Place on a lettuce leaf.

Nutrition: Calories: 330 Cal Total Fat: 26 g Saturated Fat: 0 g Cholesterol: 0mg Sodium: 0 mg Total Carbs: 3 g Fibre: 0 g Sugar: 0 g Protein: 23 g

Grilled steak

Preparation Time: 8 minutes

Cooking Time: 17 minutes

Servings: 6

Ingredients:

- A single clove of garlic
- A single tablespoon of oregano (fresh)
- ½ of a teaspoon of salt
- Four tablespoons of oil (olive)
- ¼ of a teaspoon of pepper
- ¼ of a teaspoon of pepper flakes (red ones)
- A single tablespoon of lime juice (fresh)
- Three diced avocados
- Three tablespoons of vinegar (used red wine)

What you need for the meat:

- 2 pounds of flank steak
- Pepper for seasoning
- Salt for seasoning

Directions:

1. Heat a grill to medium-high heat or 400 degrees.
2. Add all of the ingredients for the sauce to a food processor and blend until everything is smooth.
3. Get yourself a bowl.
4. Add the avocado and the sauce you blended.
5. Toss lightly, so it gets coated but not hard enough to crush the avocado.
6. Take a room temperature flank steak and season both sides with pepper and salt.
7. Remove from your grill and let cool for a few minutes.
8. Slice the steak and drizzle the top with sauce or serve it on the side.

Nutrition:

Calories: 444 Cal Total Fat: 32 g Saturated Fat: 0 g Cholesterol: 0mg Sodium: 0 mg Total Carbs: 7 g Fibre: 5 g Sugar: 0 g Protein: 34 g

Crab Chaffles

Preparation Time: 10 minutes

Cooking Time: 25 minutes

Servings: 6

Ingredients:

- 1 lb crab meat
- 1/3 cup Panko breadcrumbs
- One egg
- 2 tbsp fat greek yoghurt
- 1 tsp Dijon mustard
- 2 tbsp parsley and chives, fresh
- 1 tsp Italian seasoning
- One lemon, juiced
- Salt, pepper to taste

Directions:

1. Preheat, the waffle maker
2. Mix all the ingredients in a small mixing bowl, except crab meat.

3. Add the meat. Mix well.

4. Form the mixture into round patties.

5. Cook 1 patty for 3 minutes

6. Remove it and repeat the process with the remaining crab chaffle mixture.

7. Once ready, remove and enjoy warm.

Nutrition:

Calories: 99 Cal Total Fat: 8 g Saturated Fat: 0 g Cholesterol: 0

mg Sodium: 0 mg Total Carbs: 4 g Fibre: 0 g Sugar: 0 g Protein: 16 g

Protein Chaffles

Preparation Time: 3 minutes

Cooking Time: 4 minutes

Servings: 1

Ingredients:

- ¼ cup almond milk
- ¼ cup plant-based protein powder
- 2 tbsp almond butter
- 1 tbsp psyllium husk

Directions:

1. Preheat the waffle maker.
2. Combine almond milk, protein powder, psyllium husk, and mix thoroughly until the mixture gets the form of a paste.
3. Add in butter, combine well and form round balls
4. Place the ball in the center of the preheated waffle maker.
5. Cook for 4 minutes.
6. Remove, top as prefer and enjoy.

Nutrition:

Calories: 310 Cal Total Fat: 19 g Saturated Fat: 0 g Cholesterol: 0mg Sodium: 0 mg Total Carbs5 0 g Fibre: 0 g Sugar: 0 g Protein: 25 g

Turnip Hash Brown Chaffles

Preparation time: 10 minutes

Cooking time: 42 minutes

Servings: 6

Ingredients:

- 1 large turnip, peeled and shredded
- ½ medium white onion, minced
- 2 garlic cloves, pressed
- 1 cup finely grated Gouda cheese
- 2 eggs, beaten
- Salt and freshly ground black pepper to taste

Directions:

1. Pour the turnips in a medium safe microwave bowl, sprinkle with 1 tbsp of water, and steam in the microwave until softened, 1 to 2 minutes.
2. Remove the bowl and mix in the remaining ingredients except for a quarter cup of the Gouda cheese.
3. Preheat the waffle iron.

4. Once heated, open and sprinkle some of the reserved cheese in the iron and top with 3 tablespoons of the mixture. Close the waffle iron and cook until crispy, 5 minutes.
5. Open the lid, flip the chaffle and cook further for 2 more minutes.
6. Remove the chaffle onto a plate and set aside.
7. Make five more chaffles with the remaining batter in the same proportion.
8. Allow cooling and serve afterward.

Nutrition:

Calories: 99 Cal Total Fat: 8 g Saturated Fat: 0 g Cholesterol: 0mg Sodium: 0 mg Total Carbs: 4 g

Everything Bagel Chaffles

Preparation time: 10 minutes

Cooking time: 28 minutes

Servings: 4

Ingredients:

- 1 egg, beaten
- ½ cup finely grated Parmesan cheese
- 1 tsp Everything Bagel seasoning

Directions:

1. Preheat the waffle iron.
2. In a medium bowl, mix all the ingredients.
3. Open the iron, pour in a quarter of the mixture, close, and cook until crispy, 6 to 7 minutes.
4. Remove the chaffle onto a plate and set aside.
5. Make three more chaffles, allow cooling, and enjoy after.

Nutrition:

Calories: 99 Cal Total Fat: 8 g Saturated Fat: 0 g Cholesterol: 0mg Sodium: 0 mg Total Carbs: 4 g

Blueberry Shortcake Chaffles

Preparation time: 10 minutes

Cooking time: 14 minutes

Servings: 2

Ingredients:

- 1 egg, beaten
- 1 tbsp cream cheese, softened
- ¼ cup finely grated mozzarella cheese
- 1/4 tsp baking powder
- 4 fresh blueberries
- 1 tsp blueberry extract

Directions:

1. Preheat the waffle iron.
2. In a medium bowl, mix all the ingredients.
3. Open the iron, pour in half of the batter, close, and cook until crispy, 6 to 7 minutes.
4. Remove the chaffle onto a plate and set aside.
5. Make the other chaffle with the remaining batter.
6. Allow cooling and enjoy after.

Nutrition:

Calories: 99 Cal Total Fat: 8 g Saturated Fat: 0 g Cholesterol: 0mg Sodium: 0 mg Total Carbs: 4 g

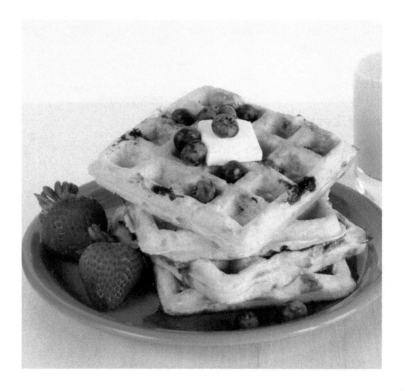

Raspberry-Pecan Chaffles

Preparation time: 10 minutes

Cooking time: 14 minutes

Servings: 2

Ingredients:

- 1 egg, beaten
- ½ cup finely grated mozzarella cheese
- 1 tbsp cream cheese, softened
- 1 tbsp sugar-free maple syrup
- ¼ tsp raspberry extract
- ¼ tsp vanilla extract
- 2 tbsp sugar-free caramel sauce for topping
- 3 tbsp chopped pecans for topping

Directions:

1. Preheat the waffle iron.
2. In a medium bowl, mix all the ingredients.
3. Open the iron, pour in half of the batter, close, and cook until crispy, 6 to 7 minutes.
4. Remove the chaffle onto a plate and set aside.

5. Make another chaffle with the remaining batter.
6. To serve: drizzle the caramel sauce on the chaffles and top with the pecans.

Nutrition:

Calories: 99 Cal Total Fat: 8 g Saturated Fat: 0 g Cholesterol: 0mg Sodium: 0 mg Total Carbs: 3 g

Scrambled Egg Stuffed Chaffles

Preparation time: 15 minutes

Cooking time: 28 minutes

Servings: 4

Ingredients:

For the chaffles:

- 1 cup finely grated cheddar cheese
- 2 eggs, beaten
- **For the egg stuffing:**
- 1 tbsp olive oil
- 4 large eggs
- 1 small green bell pepper, deseeded and chopped
- 1 small red bell pepper, deseeded and chopped
- Salt and freshly ground black pepper to taste
- 2 tbsp grated Parmesan cheese

Directions:

For the chaffles:

1. Preheat the waffle iron.

2. In a medium bowl, mix the cheddar cheese and egg.

3. Open the iron, pour in a quarter of the mixture, close, and cook until crispy, 6 to 7 minutes.

4. Plate and make three more chaffles using the remaining mixture.

For the egg stuffing:

5. Meanwhile, heat the olive oil in a medium skillet over medium heat on a stovetop.

6. In a medium bowl, beat the eggs with the bell peppers, salt, black pepper, and Parmesan cheese.

7. Pour the mixture into the skillet and scramble until set to your likeness, 2 minutes.

8. Between two chaffles, spoon half of the scrambled eggs and repeat with the second set of chaffles.

9. Serve afterward.

Nutrition:

Calories: 99 Cal Total Fat: 8 g Saturated Fat: 0 g Cholesterol: 0mg Sodium: 0 mg Total Carbs: 4 g

Mixed Berry-Vanilla Chaffles

Preparation time: 10 minutes

Cooking time: 28 minutes

Servings: 4

Ingredients:

- 1 egg, beaten
- ½ cup finely grated mozzarella cheese
- 1 tbsp cream cheese, softened
- 1 tbsp sugar-free maple syrup
- 2 strawberries, sliced
- 2 raspberries, slices
- ¼ tsp blackberry extract
- ¼ tsp vanilla extract
- ½ cup plain yogurt for serving

Directions:

1. Preheat the waffle iron.
2. In a medium bowl, mix all the ingredients except the yogurt.

3. Open the iron, lightly grease with cooking spray and pour in a quarter of the mixture.
4. Close the iron and cook until golden brown and crispy, 7 minutes.
5. Remove the chaffle onto a plate and set aside.
6. Make three more chaffles with the remaining mixture.
7. To serve: top with the yogurt and enjoy.

Nutrition:

Calories: 99 Cal Total Fat: 8 g Saturated Fat: 0 g Cholesterol: 0mg Sodium: 0 mg Total Carbs: 4 g

Ham and Cheddar Chaffles

Preparation time: 15 minutes

Cooking time: 28 minutes

Servings: 4

Ingredients:

- 1 cup finely shredded parsnips, steamed
- 8 oz ham, diced
- 2 eggs, beaten
- 1 ½ cups finely grated cheddar cheese
- ½ tsp garlic powder
- 2 tbsp chopped fresh parsley leaves
- ¼ tsp smoked paprika
- ½ tsp dried thyme
- Salt and freshly ground black pepper to taste

Directions:

1. Preheat the waffle iron.
2. In a medium bowl, mix all the ingredients.
3. Open the iron, lightly grease with cooking spray and pour in a quarter of the mixture.

4. Close the iron and cook until crispy, 7 minutes.

5. Remove the chaffle onto a plate and set aside.

6. Make three more chaffles using the remaining mixture.

7. Serve afterward.

Nutrition:

Calories: 99 Cal Total Fat: 8 g Saturated Fat: 0 g Cholesterol: 0mg Sodium: 0 mg Total Carbs: 4 g

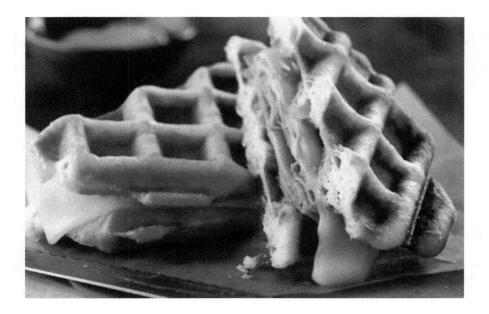

Savory Gruyere and Chives Chaffles

Preparation time: 15 minutes

Cooking time: 14 minutes

Servings: 2

Ingredients:

- 2 eggs, beaten
- 1 cup finely grated Gruyere cheese
- 2 tbsp finely grated cheddar cheese
- 1/8 tsp freshly ground black pepper
- 3 tbsp minced fresh chives + more for garnishing
- 2 sunshine fried eggs for topping

Directions:

- Preheat the waffle iron.
- In a medium bowl, mix the eggs, cheeses, black pepper, and chives.
- Open the iron and pour in half of the mixture.

- Close the iron and cook until brown and crispy, 7 minutes.
- Remove the chaffle onto a plate and set aside.
- Make another chaffle using the remaining mixture.
- Top each chaffle with one fried egg each, garnish with the chives and serve.

Nutrition:

Calories: 99 Cal Total Fat: 8 g Saturated Fat: 0 g Cholesterol: 0mg Sodium: 0 mg Total Carbs: 4 g

Chicken Quesadilla Chaffle

Preparation time: 10 minutes

Cooking time: 14 minutes

Servings: 2

Ingredients:

- 1 egg, beaten
- ¼ tsp taco seasoning
- 1/3 cup finely grated cheddar cheese
- 1/3 cup cooked chopped chicken

Directions:

1. Preheat the waffle iron.
2. In a medium bowl, mix the eggs, taco seasoning, and cheddar cheese. Add the chicken and combine well.
3. Open the iron, lightly grease with cooking spray and pour in half of the mixture.
4. Close the iron and cook until brown and crispy, 7 minutes.
5. Remove the chaffle onto a plate and set aside.
6. Make another chaffle using the remaining mixture.

7. Serve afterward.

Nutrition:

Calories: 99 Cal Total Fat: 8 g Saturated Fat: 0 g Cholesterol: 0mg Sodium: 0 mg Total Carbs: 4 g

Hot Chocolate Breakfast Chaffle

Preparation time: 10 minutes

Cooking time: 14 minutes

Servings: 2

Ingredients:

- 1 egg, beaten
- 2 tbsp almond flour
- 1 tbsp unsweetened cocoa powder
- 2 tbsp cream cheese, softened
- ¼ cup finely grated Monterey Jack cheese
- 2 tbsp sugar-free maple syrup
- 1 tsp vanilla extract

Directions:

1. Preheat the waffle iron.
2. In a medium bowl, mix all the ingredients.
3. Open the iron, lightly grease with cooking spray and pour in half of the mixture.
4. Close the iron and cook until crispy, 7 minutes.
5. Remove the chaffle onto a plate and set aside.

6. Pour the remaining batter in the iron and make the second chaffle.

7. Allow cooling and serve afterward.

Nutrition:

Calories: 99 Cal Total Fat: 8 g Saturated Fat: 0 g Cholesterol: 0mg Sodium: 0 mg Total Carbs: 2 g

Mini Breakfast Chaffles

Preparation Time: 10 minutes

Servings:3

Cooking Time: 15 Minutes

Ingredients:

- 6 tsp coconut flour
- 1 tsp stevia
- 1/4 tsp baking powder
- 2 eggs
- 3 oz. cream cheese
- 1/2. tsp vanilla extract

Topping

- 1 egg
- 6 slice bacon
- 2 oz. Raspberries for topping
- 2 oz. Blueberries for topping
- 2 oz. Strawberries for topping

Directions:

1. Heat up your square waffle maker and grease with cooking spray.
2. Mix together coconut flour, stevia, egg, baking powder, cheese and vanilla in mixing bowl.
3. Pour ½ of chaffles mixture in a waffle maker.
4. Close the lid and cook the chaffles for about 3-5 minutes Utes.
5. Meanwhile, fry bacon slices in pan on medium heat for about 2-3 minutes Utes until cooked and transfer them to plate.
6. In the same pan, fry eggs one by one in the leftover grease of bacon.
7. Once chaffles are cooked, carefully transfer them to plate.
8. Serve with fried eggs and bacon slice and berries on top.
9. Enjoy!

Nutrition:

Protein: 16% 75 kcal Fat: 75% 346 kcal Carbohydrates: 9% 41 kcal

Crispy Chaffles With Egg & Asparagus

Preparation Time: 10 minutes

Servings:1

Cooking Time: 10 Minutes

Ingredients:

- 1 egg
- 1/4 cup cheddar cheese
- 2 tbsps. almond flour
- ½ tsp. baking powder

TOPPING

- 1 egg
- 4-5 stalks asparagus
- 1 tsp avocado oil

Directions:

1. Preheat waffle maker to medium-high heat.

2. Whisk together egg, mozzarella cheese, almond flour, and baking powder

3. Pour chaffles mixture into the center of the waffle iron. Close the waffle maker and let cook for 5 minutes Utes or until waffle is golden brown and set.

4. Remove chaffles from the waffle maker and serve.

5. Meanwhile, heat oil in a nonstick pan.

6. Once the pan is hot, fry asparagus for about 4-5 minutes Utes until golden brown.

7. Poach the egg in boil water for about 2-3 minutes Utes.

8. Once chaffles are cooked, remove from the maker.

9. Serve chaffles with the poached egg and asparagus.

Nutrition:

Protein: 26% 85 kcal Fat: 69% 226 kcal Carbohydrates: 5% 16 kcal

Delicious Raspberries taco Chaffles

Preparation Time: 10 minutes

Servings:1

Cooking Time: 15 Minutes

Ingredients:

- 1 egg white
- 1/4 cup jack cheese, shredded
- 1/4 cup cheddar cheese, shredded
- 1 tsp coconut flour
- 1/4 tsp baking powder
- 1/2 tsp stevia

For Topping

- 4 oz. raspberries
- 2 tbsps. coconut flour
- 2 oz. unsweetened raspberry sauce

Directions:

1. Switch on your round Waffle Maker and grease it with cooking spray once it is hot.
2. Mix together all chaffle ingredients in a bowl and combine with a fork.
3. Pour chaffle batter in a preheated maker and close the lid.
4. Roll the taco chaffle around using a kitchen roller, set it aside and allow it to set for a few minutes Utes.
5. Once the taco chaffle is set, remove from the roller.
6. Dip raspberries in sauce and arrange on taco chaffle.
7. Drizzle coconut flour on top.
8. Enjoy raspberries taco chaffle with keto coffee.

Nutrition:

Protein: 28% 77 kcal Fat: 6 187 kcal Carbohydrates: 3% 8 kcal

Coconut Chaffles

Preparation Time: 10 minutes

Servings:2

Cooking Time: 5 Minutes

Ingredients:

- 1 egg
- 1 oz. cream cheese,
- 1 oz. cheddar cheese
- 2 tbsps. coconut flour
- 1 tsp. stevia
- 1 tbsp. coconut oil, melted
- 1/2 tsp. coconut extract
- 2 eggs, soft boil for serving

Directions:

1. Heat you minutes Dash waffle maker and grease with cooking spray.
2. Mix together all chaffles ingredients in a bowl.
3. Pour chaffle batter in a preheated waffle maker.

4. Close the lid.

5. Cook chaffles for about 2-3 minutes Utes until golden brown.

6. Serve with boil egg and enjoy!

Nutrition:

Protein: 21% 32 kcal Fat: % 117 kcal Carbohydrates: 3% 4 kcal

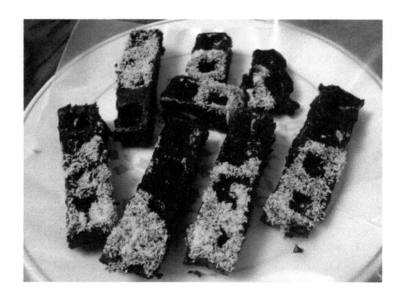

Garlic and Parsley Chaffles

Preparation Time: 10 minutes

Servings:1

Cooking Time: 5 Minutes

Ingredients:

- 1 large egg
- 1/4 cup cheese mozzarella
- 1 tsp. coconut flour
- ¼ tsp. baking powder
- ½ tsp. garlic powder
- 1 tbsp. minutes parsley

For Serving

- 1 Poach egg
- 4 oz. smoked salmon

Directions:

1. Switch on your Dash minutes waffle maker and let it preheat.

2. Grease waffle maker with cooking spray.

3. Mix together egg, mozzarella, coconut flour, baking powder, and garlic powder, parsley to a mixing bowl until combined well.

4. Pour batter in circle chaffle maker.

5. Close the lid.

6. Cook for about 2-3 minutes Utes or until the chaffles are cooked.

7. Serve with smoked salmon and poached egg.

8. Enjoy!

Nutrition:

Protein: 45% 140 kcal Fat: 51% 160 kcal Carbohydrates: 4% 14 kcal

Scrambled Eggs on A Spring Onion Chaffle

Preparation Time: 10 minutes

Servings:4

Cooking Time:7–9 Minutes

Ingredients:

- Batter
- 4 eggs
- 2 cups grated mozzarella cheese
- 2 spring onions, finely chopped
- Salt and pepper to taste
- ½ teaspoon dried garlic powder
- 2 tablespoons almond flour
- 2 tablespoons coconut flour

Other

- 2 tablespoons butter for brushing the waffle maker
- 6-8 eggs
- Salt and pepper
- 1 teaspoon Italian spice mix
- 1 tablespoon olive oil

- 1 tablespoon freshly chopped parsley

Directions:

1. Preheat the waffle maker.
2. Crack the eggs into a bowl and add the grated cheese.
3. Mix until just combined, then add the chopped spring onions and season with salt and pepper and dried garlic powder.
4. Stir in the almond flour and mix until everything is combined.
5. Brush the heated waffle maker with butter and add a few tablespoons of the batter.
6. Close the lid and cook for about 7–8 minutes depending on your waffle maker.
7. While the chaffles are cooking, prepare the scrambled eggs by whisking the eggs in a bowl until frothy, about 2 minutes. Season with salt and black pepper to taste and add the Italian spice mix. Whisk to blend in the spices.
8. Warm the oil in a non-stick pan over medium heat.
9. Pour the eggs in the pan and cook until eggs are set to your liking.
10. Serve each chaffle and top with some scrambled eggs. Top with freshly chopped parsley.

Nutrition:

Calories 194 Fat 14.7 g, carbs 5 g, sugar 0.6 g, Protein   1   g, sodium 191 mg

Egg on A Cheddar Cheese Chaffle

Preparation Time: 10 minutes

Servings:4

Cooking Time:7–9 Minutes

Ingredients:

Batter

- 4 eggs
- 2 cups shredded white cheddar cheese
- Salt and pepper to taste

Other

- 2 tablespoons butter for brushing the waffle maker
- 4 large eggs
- 2 tablespoons olive oil

Directions:

1. Preheat the waffle maker.
2. Crack the eggs into a bowl and whisk them with a fork.

3. Stir in the grated cheddar cheese and season with salt and pepper.
4. Brush the heated waffle maker with butter and add a few tablespoons of the batter.
5. Close the lid and cook for about 7–8 minutes depending on your waffle maker.
6. While chaffles are cooking, cook the eggs.
7. Warm the oil in a large non-stick pan that has a lid over medium-low heat for 2-3 minutes
8. Crack an egg in a small ramekin and gently add it to the pan. Repeat the same way for the other 3 eggs.
9. Cover and let cook for 2 to 2 ½ minutes for set eggs but with runny yolks.
10. Remove from heat.
11. To serve, place a chaffle on each plate and top with an egg. Season with salt and black pepper to taste.

Nutrition:

Calories 4 fat 34 g, carbs 2 g, sugar 0.6 g, Protein 26 g, sodium 518 mg

Avocado Chaffle Toast

Preparation Time: 10 minutes

Servings:3

Cooking Time: 10 Minutes

Ingredients:

- 4 tbsps. avocado mash
- 1/2 tsp lemon juice
- 1/8 tsp salt
- 1/8 tsp black pepper
- 2 eggs
- 1/2 cup shredded cheese

For serving

- 3 eggs
- ½ avocado thinly sliced
- 1 tomato, sliced

Directions:

1. Mash avocado mash with lemon juice, salt, and black pepper in mixing bowl, until well combined.
2. In a small bowl beat egg and pour eggs in avocado mixture and mix well.
3. Switch on Waffle Maker to pre-heat.
4. Pour 1/8 of shredded cheese in a waffle maker and then pour ½ of egg and avocado mixture and then 1/8 shredded cheese.
5. Close the lid and cook chaffles for about 3 - 4 minutes Utes.
6. Repeat with the remaining mixture.
7. Meanwhile, fry eggs in a pan for about 1-2 minutes Utes.
8. For serving, arrange fried egg on chaffle toast with avocado slice and tomatoes.
9. Sprinkle salt and pepper on top and enjoy!

Nutrition:

Protein: 26% 66 kcal Fat: 67% 169 kcal Carbohydrates: 6% 15kcal

Cajun & Feeta Chaffles

Preparation Time: 10 minutes

Servings:1

Cooking Time: 10 Minutes

Ingredients:

- 1 egg white
- 1/4 cup shredded mozzarella cheese
- 2 tbsps. almond flour
- 1 tsp Cajun Seasoning

FOR SERVING

- 1 egg
- 4 oz. feta cheese
- 1 tomato, sliced

Directions:

1. Whisk together egg, cheese, and seasoning in a bowl.
2. Switch on and grease waffle maker with cooking spray.
3. Pour batter in a preheated waffle maker.

4. Cook chaffles for about 2-3 minutes Utes until the chaffle is cooked through.
5. Meanwhile, fry the egg in a non-stick pan for about 1-2 minutes Utes.
6. For serving set fried egg on chaffles with feta cheese and tomatoes slice.

Nutrition:

Protein: 28% 119 kcal Fat: 64% 2 kcal Carbohydrates: 7% 31 kcal

Crispy Chaffles With Sausage

Preparation Time: 10 minutes

Servings:2

Cooking Time: 10 Minutes

Ingredients:

- 1/2 cup cheddar cheese
- 1/2 tsp. baking powder
- 1/4 cup egg whites
- 2 tsp. pumpkin spice
- 1 egg, whole
- 2 chicken sausage
- 2 slice bacon
- salt and pepper to taste
- 1 tsp. avocado oil

Directions:

1. Mix together all ingredients in a bowl.
2. Allow batter to sit while waffle iron warms.
3. Spray waffle iron with nonstick spray.

4. Pour batter in the waffle maker and cook according to the directions of the manufacturer.
5. Meanwhile, heat oil in a pan and fry the egg, according to your choice and transfer it to plate.
6. In the same pan, fry bacon slice and sausage on medium heat for about 2-3 minutes Utes until cooked.
7. Once chaffles are cooked thoroughly, remove them from the maker.
8. Serve with fried egg, bacon slice, sausages and enjoy!

Nutrition:

Protein: 22% 86 kcal Fat: 74% 286 kcal Carbohydrates: 3% 12 kcal

Chili Chaffle

Preparation Time: 10 minutes

Servings:4

Cooking Time:7–9 Minutes

Ingredients:

Batter

- 4 eggs
- ½ cup grated parmesan cheese
- 1½ cups grated yellow cheddar cheese
- 1 hot red chili pepper
- Salt and pepper to taste
- ½ teaspoon dried garlic powder
- 1 teaspoon dried basil
- 2 tablespoons almond flour

Other

- 2 tablespoons olive oil for brushing the waffle maker

Directions:

1. Preheat the waffle maker.
2. Crack the eggs into a bowl and add the grated parmesan and cheddar cheese.
3. Mix until just combined and add the chopped chili pepper. Season with salt and pepper, dried garlic powder and dried basil. Stir in the almond flour.
4. Mix until everything is combined.
5. Brush the heated waffle maker with olive oil and add a few tablespoons of the batter.
6. Close the lid and cook for about 7–8 minutes depending on your waffle maker.

Nutrition:

Calories 36 fat 30.4 g, carbs 3.1 g, sugar 0.7 g, Protein 21.5 g, sodium 469 mg

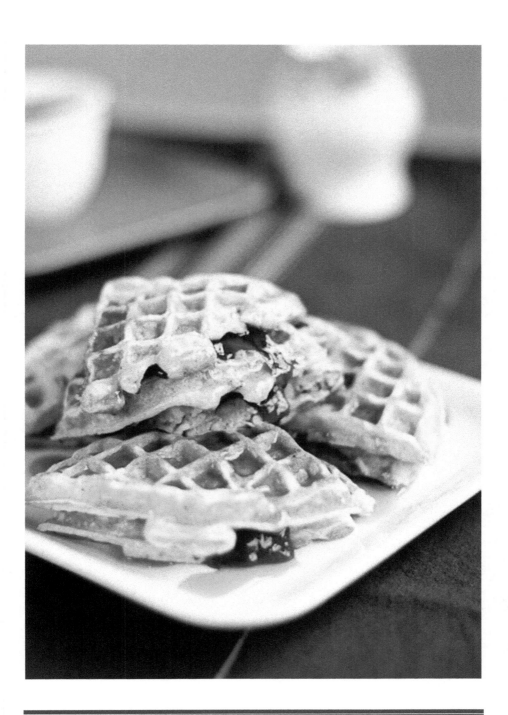